Vegetarian Sweet Secrets

50 Sweet Easy-to-Make Delicious Recipes for Your Vegetarian Treats & Desserts

Kaylee Collins

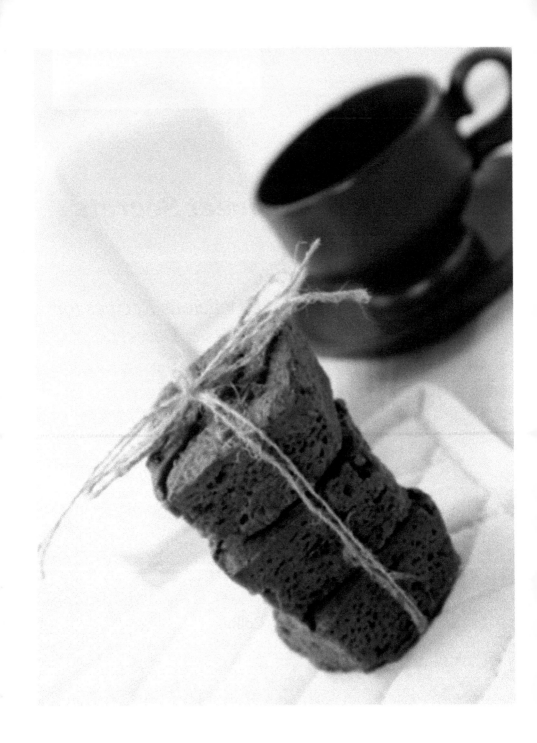

Table of Contents

Chocolate Chip Mini Muffins

Prep time: 5 min Cooking Time: 20 min serve: 2

Ingredients

½ cup coconut flour

1 egg

½ cup sugar-free chocolate chips

½ tablespoon vanilla extract

½ cup honey

1 tablespoon coconut

¼ teaspoon salt

¼ teaspoon baking soda

Instructions

Pour 1 cup of filtered water into the Instant Pot's inner pot, then insert the trivet. Using an electric mixer, combine coconut flour, egg, chocolate chips, vanilla, honey, coconut, salt, and baking soda. Mix thoroughly.

Using a sling if desired, place the pan onto the trivet and cover loosely with aluminium foil. Close the lid, set the Pressure Release to Sealing, and select Manual/Pressure Cook. Set the Instant Pot to 20 minutes on High Pressure and let cook.

Once cooked, let the pressure release naturally from the Instant Pot for about 10 minutes, then carefully switch the Pressure Release to Venting.

Open the Instant Pot and remove the pan. Let cool, serve and enjoy!

Nutrition Facts

Calories 366, Total Fat 4.8g, Saturated Fat 2.3g, Cholesterol 82mg, Sodium 508mg, Total Carbohydrate 76.8g, Dietary Fiber 1.7g , Total Sugars 70.6g, Protein 3.9g

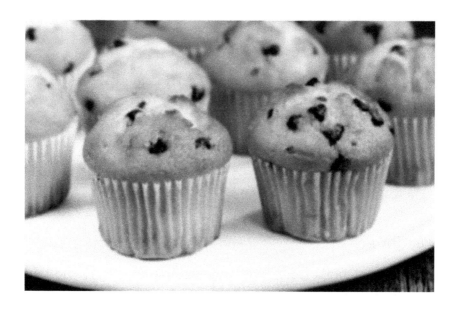

Pumpkin Spice Coffee Muffins

Prep time: 5 min Cooking Time: 20 min serve: 2

Ingredients

1/4 tablespoon coffee

1 cup coconut flour

2 tablespoons honey

½ cup pumpkin puree

1 tablespoon coconut oil

1 egg

1 teaspoon baking soda

¼ teaspoon ground allspice

½ teaspoon baking powder

1 tablespoon chocolate chips

Directions

In the instant pot's inner pot, put water then insert the trivet. Combine warm water and coffee in a cup until coffee is dissolved; pour into a large bowl. Mix coconut flour, honey, pumpkin puree, coconut oil, egg, baking soda, salt, allspice, and baking powder into coffee until batter is thoroughly mixed; fold in chocolate chips. Fill muffin cups with batter.

Using a sling if desired, place the pan onto the trivet and cover loosely with aluminium foil. Close the lid, set the Pressure Release to Sealing, and select Manual/Pressure Cook. Set the Instant Pot to 20 minutes on High Pressure and let cook.

Once cooked, let the pressure release naturally from the Instant Pot for about 10 minutes, then carefully switch the Pressure Release to Venting.

Open the Instant Pot and remove the pan. Let cool, serve and enjoy!

Nutrition Facts

Calories 235, Total Fat 11.8g, Saturated Fat 8.8g, Cholesterol 83mg, Sodium 1266mg, Total Carbohydrate 30.3g, Dietary Fiber 4.6g, Total Sugars 22.6g, Protein 4.9g

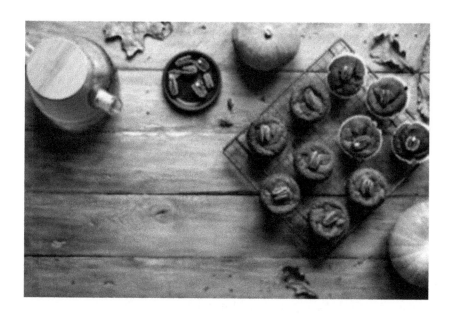

Blueberry Cream Muffins

Prep time: 10 min Cooking Time: 20 min serve: 2

Ingredients

1 egg

2 tablespoons maple syrup

1 tablespoon coconut oil

½ teaspoon vanilla extract

½ cup coconut flour

½ teaspoon salt

½ teaspoon baking soda

2 tablespoons coconut cream

2 tablespoons blueberries

Instructions

Grease 4 muffin cups or line with paper muffin liners. In large bowl beat egg, gradually add maple syrup while beating. Continue beating while slowly pouring in oil. Stir in vanilla. In a separate bowl, stir together flour, salt and baking soda.

Stir dry ingredients into egg mixture alternately with coconut cream. Gently fold in blueberries. Scoop batter into prepared muffin cups. Place the pan onto the trivet and cover loosely with aluminium foil. Close the lid, set the Pressure Release to Sealing, and select Manual/Pressure Cook. Set the Instant Pot to 20 minutes on High Pressure and let cook.

Once cooked, let the pressure release naturally from the Instant Pot for about 10 minutes, then carefully switch the Pressure Release to Venting.

Open the Instant Pot and remove the pan. Let cool, serve and enjoy!

Nutrition Facts

Calories 215, Total Fat 13.6g, Saturated Fat 10.7g, Cholesterol 82mg, Sodium 946mg, Total Carbohydrate 19.9g, Dietary Fiber 3.1g, Total Sugars 14.1g , Protein 4.2g

Apple Pumpkin Muffins

Prep time: 15 min Cooking Time: 20 min serve: 2

Ingredients

½ cup almond flour

¼ cup coconut flour

½ cup honey

¼ tablespoon pumpkin pie spice

¼ teaspoon baking soda

¼ teaspoon salt

1 egg

1 tablespoon pumpkin puree

½ tablespoon coconut oil

½ cup peeled and chopped apples

3 tablespoons butter, softened

½ tablespoon maple syrup

¼ cup wheat flour

1 teaspoon ground cinnamon

Instructions

Combine coconut flour, almond flour, honey, pumpkin pie spice, baking soda, and salt in a large bowl. Mix egg, pumpkin, and coconut oil in a small bowl. Stir egg mixture into flour mixture until just moistened; fold in apples. Fill prepared muffin cups 2/3 full.

Combine butter, ½ cup maple syrup, ¼ cup whole wheat flour, and cinnamon in a small bowl; sprinkle over muffin batter.

Place the pan onto the trivet and cover loosely with aluminium foil. Close

the lid, set the Pressure Release to Sealing, and select Manual/Pressure Cook. Set the Instant Pot to 20 minutes on High Pressure and let cook.

Once cooked, let the pressure release naturally from the Instant Pot for about 10 minutes, then carefully switch the Pressure Release to Venting.

Open the Instant Pot and remove the pan. Let cool, serve and enjoy!

Nutrition Facts

Calories 383, Total Fat 18.7g, Saturated Fat 8g, Cholesterol 64mg, Sodium 308mg, Total Carbohydrate

48.2g, Dietary Fiber 3.2g , Total Sugars 37.7g, Protein 5.6g

Pineapple Zucchini Muffins

Prep time: 30 min Cooking Time: 20 min serve: 2

Ingredients

½ cup coconut flour

½ tablespoon maple syrup

¼ teaspoon baking powder

½ teaspoon baking soda

½ teaspoon ground cinnamon

1tablespoon coconut oil

1 egg

3 tablespoons shredded zucchini

1 tablespoon crushed pineapple, drained

½ teaspoon vanilla extract

Instructions

In a large bowl, combine coconut flour, maple syrup, baking powder, baking soda, cinnamon and salt. Make a well in the centre, and pour in the oil, egg, zucchini, pineapple and vanilla. Mix until smooth. Fill muffin cups 2/3 to 3/4 packed.

Place the pan onto the trivet and cover loosely with aluminium foil. Close the lid, set the Pressure Release to Sealing, and select Manual/Pressure Cook. Set the Instant Pot to 20 minutes on High Pressure and let cook.

Once cooked, let the pressure release naturally from the Instant Pot for about 10 minutes, then carefully switch the Pressure Release to Venting.

Open the Instant Pot and remove the pan. Let cool, serve and enjoy!

Nutrition Facts

Calories 64, Total Fat 4.8g, Saturated Fat 3.5g, Cholesterol 41mg, Sodium 470mg, Total Carbohydrate 3.7g, Dietary Fiber 0.9g, Total Sugars 2.1g, Protein 1.7g

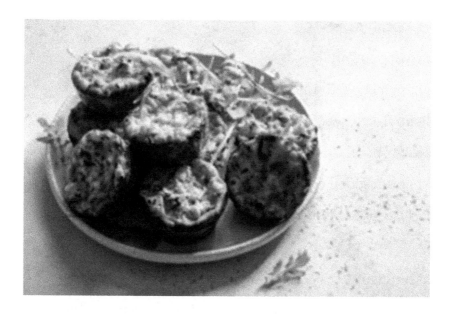

Carrot Oatmeal Muffins

Prep time: 30 min Cooking Time: 20 min serve: 2

Ingredients

½ cup almond flour

¼ cup coconut flour

½ teaspoons baking soda

½ teaspoon baking powder

¼ teaspoon salt

¼ teaspoon cinnamon

1 tablespoon honey

1 cup coconut oil

1 egg, beaten

½ teaspoon vanilla extract

¼ cup uncooked rolled oats

¼ cup flaked coconut

½ tablespoon raisins

½ cup shredded carrots

¼ cup crushed pineapple

Instructions

In a large bowl, mix the almond flour, coconut flour, baking soda, baking powder, salt, and cinnamon. Make a well in the centre of the mixture, and add honey, coconut oil, egg, and vanilla. Mix just until evenly moist. Fold in the oats, coconut flour, raisins, carrots, and pineapple.

Fill each muffin cup is about 2/3 full.

Place the pan onto the trivet and cover loosely with aluminium foil. Close the lid, set the Pressure Release to Sealing, and select Manual/Pressure Cook. Set the Instant Pot to 20 minutes on High Pressure and let cook.

Once cooked, let the pressure release naturally from the Instant Pot for about 10 minutes, then carefully switch the Pressure Release to Venting.

Open the Instant Pot and remove the pan. Let cool, serve and enjoy!

Nutrition Facts

Calories 379, Total Fat 22.8g, Saturated Fat 6.9g, Cholesterol 82mg , Sodium 664mg, Total Carbohydrate 32.4g, Dietary Fiber 6.8g, Total Sugars 15.5g, Protein 11.2g

Banana Blueberry Muffins

Prep time: 30 min Cooking Time: 20 min serve: 2

Ingredients

½ cup flax meal

½ tablespoon honey

1/8 teaspoon ground cinnamon

¼ teaspoons baking powder

¼ teaspoon baking soda

1 mashed banana

1 egg white

1/8 teaspoon vanilla extract

1 tablespoon fresh blueberries

1 cup water

Instructions

Mix the flax meal, honey, cinnamon, baking powder, and baking soda. In a separate bowl, mix the banana, egg white, and vanilla extract.

Mix the banana mixture into the flour mixture until smooth. Fold in the blueberries. Spoon the batter into the pan prepared for the muffins.

Pour 1 cup water into the Instant Pot. Place the trivet inside. Place the muffin cups on the rack or pan.

Secure the lid and set the Pressure Release valve to Sealing. Press the Pressure Cook or Manual button and set the cook time to 20 minutes.

When the Instant Pot beeps, allow the pressure to release naturally for 10 minutes, then carefully switch the Pressure Release valve to Venting. When fully released, open the lid. Carefully remove the muffins. Allow them to cool for about 15 minutes.

Nutrition Facts

Calories 233, Total Fat 10.2g, Saturated Fat 0.1g, Cholesterol 0mg, Sodium 177mg, Total Carbohydrate 27g, Dietary Fiber 9.7g, Total Sugars 12.1g, Protein 8.5g

Lemon Zucchini Muffins

Prep time: 15 min Cooking Time: 25 min serve: 2

Ingredients

½ cup coconut flour

2 tablespoons honey

¼ teaspoon baking powder

¼ teaspoon baking soda

1/8 teaspoon salt

½ zucchini, shredded

¼ cup lemon yogurt

2 tablespoons butter, melted

1 egg, beaten

1 tablespoon lemon juice

1 tablespoon lemon zest

1 cup water

Instructions

Mix flour, honey, baking powder, baking soda, and salt in a large bowl; make a well in the centre of the flour mixture. Mix zucchini, yogurt, butter, egg, 1 tablespoon lemon juice, and 1 tablespoon lemon zest in a separate bowl; pour yogurt mixture into well.

Pour 1 cup water into the Instant Pot. Place the trivet inside. Place the muffin cups on the rack or pan.

Secure the lid and set the Pressure Release valve to Sealing. Press the Pressure Cook or Manual button and set the cook time to 20 minutes.

When the Instant Pot beeps, allow the pressure to release naturally for 10 minutes, then carefully switch the Pressure Release valve to Venting. When fully released, open the lid. Carefully remove the muffins. Allow them to cool for about 15 minutes.

Nutrition Facts

Calories 244, Total Fat 14.7g, Saturated Fat 8.8g, Cholesterol 114mg, Sodium 455mg, Total Carbohydrate 23.8g, Dietary Fiber 1.9g, Total Sugars 20.8g, Protein 5.8g

Banana Chocolate Chip Muffins

Prep time: 15 min Cooking Time: 20 min serve: 2

Ingredients

½ cup almond flour

1 tablespoon honey

½ teaspoon cocoa powder

1/8 tablespoon baking powder

1 mashed banana

½ teaspoon olive oil

1 egg, beaten

1tablespoon semi-sweet chocolate chips

1 cup water

Instructions

In a large bowl combine the flour, honey, cocoa powder and baking powder.

In another bowl, blend the banana, oil and egg. Add to dry ingredients, mixing just until blended. Fold in the chocolate chips.

Pour 1 cup water into the Instant Pot. Place the trivet inside. Place the muffin cups on the rack or pan.

Secure the lid and set the Pressure Release valve to Sealing. Press the Pressure Cook or Manual button and set the cook time to 20 minutes.

When the Instant Pot beeps, allow the pressure to release naturally for 10 minutes, then carefully switch the Pressure Release valve to Venting. When fully released, open the lid. Carefully remove the muffins. Allow them to cool for about 15 minutes.

Nutrition Facts

Calories 189, Total Fat 10.5g, Saturated Fat 1.5g, Cholesterol 41mg, Sodium 39mg, Total Carbohydrate 18.7g, Dietary Fiber 2.6g, Total Sugars 11.2g, Protein 5g

Brownie Muffins

Servings 6

Ingredients

1 cup golden flaxseed meal

¼ cup cocoa powder

1 tablespoon cinnamon

½ tablespoon baking powder

½ teaspoon salt 1 large egg

2 tablespoons coconut oil

¼ cup sugar-free caramel syrup

½ cup pumpkin puree

1 teaspoon vanilla extract

1 teaspoon apple cider vinegar

¼ cup slivered almonds

Instructions

Preheat your oven to 350°F and combine all your dry ingredients in a deep mixing bowl and mix to combine.

In a separate bowl, combine all your wet ingredients.

Pour your wet ingredients into your dry ingredients and mix very well to combine.

Line a muffin tin with paper liners and spoon about ¼ cup of batter into each muffin liner. This recipe should Servings 6 muffins. Then sprinkle slivered almonds over the top of each muffin and press gently so that they adhere.

Bake in the oven for about 15 minutes. You should see the muffins rise and set on top. Enjoy warm or cool!

Nutrition Info

193 Calories 14.09g Fats 4.37g Net Carbs 6.98g Protein.

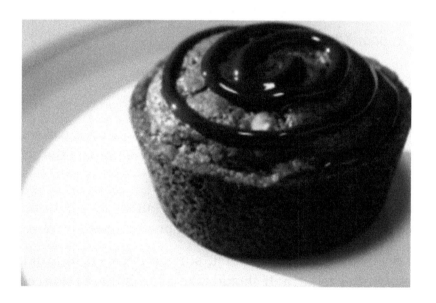

No-bake keto cookies

No-bake keto cookies aka. keto almond clusters with 1.9 grams of net carbs per serving

Prep Time: 5 mins Total Time: 15 mins 10 cookies

Ingredients

1/3 cup almond butter

1 tablespoon Coconut oil

1/2 cup Sugar-free Chocolate Chips 1 1/4 cup Sliced almonds

1 tablespoon Chia seeds

Instructions

Cover a large plate or chopping board with a piece of parchment paper. Place the plate in the freezer while you prepare the cookie batter.

In a microwave-safe bowl, add almond butter, coconut oil, and sugar-free chocolate chips (or bars chopped in small pieces).

Microwave by 30 seconds burst, stirring between to avoid the almond butter to burn. It should take a maximum of 90 seconds to fully combine all your ingredients.

If you don't have a microwave, place all the ingredients into a small saucepan. Place under medium heat and stir all the time until chocolate melt and all the ingredients are combined.

Stir in the sliced almonds and chia seeds. You want to fully cover the almonds and seeds with the chocolate mixture.

Remove the plate from the freezer.

Spoon some cookie batter, then place the batter onto the prepared cold plate covered with parchment paper. As the plate is cold, the cookie shouldn't expand too much and the base should set fast. Leave 1 thumb space between each cookie just in case they expand slightly. Repeat until no more batter left.

You should be able to form 10 bite-size cookies.

Place the plate back in the freezer for 10 minutes or until the chocolate is firm and set.

Store your cookies in an airtight container in the fridge for up to 3 weeks. They are crunchier if stored in the fridge.

You can triple the recipe to meal prep your snack for the week and freeze those cookies in a zip bag for later. Defrost for 3-4 hours before eating.

Nutrition Info

Calories 141 Calories from Fat 113 Fat 12.5g19% Carbohydrates 4.9g2% Fiber 3g13% Sugar 0.9g1% Protein 4.5g

Chocolate Avocado Cookies

Chocolate avocado cookies are healthy fudgy chocolate cookies made of 5 simple ingredients

Prep Time: 10 mins Cook Time: 12 mins Total Time: 22 mins 6 cookies

Ingredients

1 Avocado about 1/2 cup mashed avocado

1/4 cup Sugar-free flavored maple syrup or maple syrup (if not low carb)

1/2 cup Nut butter peanut butter or almond butter (if paleo) 1 Egg or chia egg if vegan

1/2 cup unsweetened cocoa powder

1/4 cup Sugar-free Chocolate Chips or choose your favorite one 1 teaspoon Vanilla extract

2-3 drops Monk Fruit Drops or Stevia Drops

Instructions

Preheat oven to 180°C (360°F)

Cover a baking sheet with parchment paper. Slightly oil the paper with 1/2 teaspoon of liquid vegetable oil (coconut or peanut oil). This will prevent the cookies to stick to the paper. Set aside.

In a food processor, with the S blade attachment, add ripe avocado and sugar-free maple syrup (or li☐uid sweetener you like). Process for 30 seconds until it forms a creamy avocado batter with no lumps.

Stop, add egg, nut butter, and cocoa powder. Process again for 30 seconds. Scrape down the bottom and side of the bowl and process for an extra 15 seconds to make sure all the batter is combined - no lumps.

Transfer the chocolate cookie batter onto a mixing bowl. It will bit moist and sticky that is what you want. Stir in chocolate chips and vanilla - if used.

Combine with a spatula until the chocolate chips are evenly incorporated. Test the batter and adjust with 2-3 drops of liquid stevia - only if you want a sweeter cookie. I did not add any to mine but if you have a sweet tooth I recommend few drops of stevia to make them sweeter. Add one drop at a time and see how it tastes.

Prepare a small bowl with warm water, dip a spoon in the water, and use that spoon to sample some chocolate cookie batter from your bowl. The water will prevent the batter to stick too much to your spoon.

Spoon the chocolate batter onto the baking sheet - I used another spoon to push the batter out of the first spoon. Use a silicone spoon or spatula to flatten the cookie into a cookie shape. The batter won't stick onto silicone which makes it easier to spread.

Repeat until you form 6 jumbo cookies. Those cookies won't spread so you don't need to leave more than half thumb space between each.

Sprinkle extra chocolate chips on top of each cookie if you like. Bake for 12-15 minutes or until the center is set.

Cool it down for 5 minutes on the baking sheet then transfer onto a cooling rack to cool down.

Store the cookies in the fridge for up to 5 days in an airtight container.

Nutrition Info

Calories 187 Calories from Fat 146 Fat 16.2g25% Carbohydrates 10.4g Fiber 4.9g20% Sugar 1.2g1% Protein 7.1g

Sweet Corn Muffins

Prep time: 10 min Cooking Time: 25 min serve: 2

Ingredients

½ cup coconut flour

1 tablespoon maple syrup

2 tablespoons cornmeal

¼ teaspoon baking powder

¼ teaspoon salt

1/8 cup sweet corn

1 egg, beaten

¼ cup applesauce

½ cup coconut milk

1 cup water

Instructions

Mix coconut flour, maple, cornmeal, baking powder, and salt in a large mixing bowl. Add sweet corn, egg, applesauce, and ¼ cup coconut milk to the flour mixture and beat with an electric hand mixer for 1 minute. Pour remaining milk into the batter and beat until just blended. Fill muffin tins 3/4 full of batter.

Pour 1 cup water into the Instant Pot. Place the trivet inside. Place the muffin cups on the rack or pan.

Secure the lid and set the Pressure Release valve to Sealing. Press the Pressure Cook or Manual button and set the cook time to 20 minutes.

When the Instant Pot beeps, allow the pressure to release naturally for 10 minutes, then carefully switch the Pressure Release valve to Venting. When fully released, open the lid. Carefully remove the muffins. Cool in the pans for 10 minutes before removing to cool completely on a wire rack.

Nutrition Facts

Calories 124, Total Fat 5.5g, Saturated Fat 3.9g, Cholesterol 41mg, Sodium 177mg, Total Carbohydrate

17.3g, Dietary Fiber 2.5g, Total Sugars 6.5g, Protein 3.6g

Blueberry Pumpkin Muffins

Prep time: 15 min Cooking Time: 20 min serve: 2

Ingredients

½ cup coconut flour

1 tablespoon quick cooking oats

1 tablespoon honey

½ teaspoon baking powder

¼ teaspoon salt

½ teaspoon ground cinnamon

½ teaspoon nutmeg

¼ cup canned pumpkin

1/8 cup coconut milk

1 egg

1/8 cup butter, melted

¼ cup fresh blueberries

1 cup water

Instructions

Mix the coconut flour, oats, honey, baking powder, salt, cinnamon, and nutmeg in a mixing bowl until evenly blended. In a separate bowl, stir together the pumpkin, coconut milk, egg, and butter. Gradually stir in the flour mixture, just until all ingredients are moistened. Fold in the blueberries.

Pour 1 cup water into the Instant Pot. Place the trivet inside. Place the muffin cups on the rack or pan.

Secure the lid and set the Pressure Release valve to Sealing. Press the Pressure Cook or Manual button and set the cook time to 20 minutes.

When the Instant Pot beeps, allow the pressure to release naturally for 10 minutes, then carefully switch the Pressure Release valve to Venting. When fully released, open the lid. Carefully remove the muffins.

Nutrition Facts

Calories 125, Total Fat 9.1g, Saturated Fat 5.9g, Cholesterol 56mg, Sodium 210mg, Total Carbohydrate

9.9g, Dietary Fiber 1.8g , Total Sugars 6.3g, Protein 2.3g

Cornmeal Quinoa Poppy Seed Muffins

Prep time: 15 min Cooking Time: 20 min serve: 2

Ingredients

½ cup quinoa flour

½ cup coconut flour

½ tablespoon yellow cornmeal

¼ teaspoon poppy seeds

1 tablespoon maple syrup

¼ tablespoon grated lemon

¼ teaspoon baking powder

½ teaspoon baking soda

Pinch salt

¼ cup coconut milk

¼ tablespoon coconut oil

1 egg

¼ teaspoon vanilla extract

1 cup water

Instructions

Mix quinoa flour, coconut flour, cornmeal, poppy seeds, maple syrup, grated lemon, baking powder, baking soda, and salt in a bowl.

Whisk coconut milk, coconut oil, egg, and vanilla extract together in a separate bowl. Stir milk mixture into flour mixture until just combined. Pour batter into the prepared muffin cups.

Pour 1 cup water into the Instant Pot. Place the trivet inside. Place the muffin cups on the rack or pan.

Secure the lid and set the Pressure Release valve to Sealing. Press the Pressure Cook or Manual button and set the cook time to 20 minutes.

When the Instant Pot beeps, allow the pressure to release naturally for 10 minutes, then carefully switch the Pressure Release valve to Venting. When fully released, open the lid. Carefully remove the muffins.

Nutrition Facts

Calories 162, Total Fat 7.2g, Saturated Fat 4.7g, Cholesterol 41mg, Sodium 221mg, Total Carbohydrate 19.9g, Dietary Fiber 2.6g, Total Sugars 3.8g, Protein 5.1g

Berry Muffins

Prep time: 15 min Cooking Time: 30 min serve: 2

Ingredients

½ cup coconut flour

1 tablespoon rolled oats

1 tablespoon honey

½ teaspoon baking powder

¼ teaspoon ground cinnamon

¼ cup coconut milk

1 egg, beaten

1 tablespoon coconut oil

½ cup fresh blueberries

1 cup water

Instructions

In a medium-size bowl, combine coconut flour, oats, honey, baking powder, and cinnamon. Stir in milk, egg, and oil. Continue stirring until the mixture is well blended. Fold in the blueberries. Spoon the mixture into the muffin cups 2/3 full.

Pour 1 cup water into the Instant Pot. Place the trivet inside. Place the muffin cups on the rack or pan.

Secure the lid and set the Pressure Release valve to Sealing. Press the Pressure Cook or Manual button and set the cook time to 20 minutes.

When the Instant Pot beeps, allow the pressure to release naturally for 10 minutes, then carefully switch the Pressure Release valve to Venting. When fully released, open the lid. Carefully remove the muffins.

Nutrition Facts

Calories 119, Total Fat 8.5g, Saturated Fat 6.7g, Cholesterol 41mg, Sodium 22mg, Total Carbohydrate

Eggplant Walnut Muffins

Prep time: 15 min Cooking Time: 30 min serve: 2

Ingredients

½ cup coconut flour

¼ teaspoon salt

¼ teaspoon ground nutmeg

¼ teaspoon baking soda

¼ teaspoon baking powder

1 egg

½ tablespoon honey

1 tablespoon coconut oil

½ cup grated eggplant

1 tablespoon walnut

1 cup water

Instructions

Mix coconut flour, salt, nutmeg, baking soda, and baking powder in a mixing bowl.

Beat egg, honey, and coconut oil together in a large bowl. Fold eggplant and walnut into egg mixture until evenly mixed. Stir flour mixture into the wet mixture to make a batter. Divide batter into muffin cups to about 2/3 full.

Pour 1 cup water into the Instant Pot. Place the trivet inside. Place the muffin cups on the rack or pan.

Secure the lid and set the Pressure Release valve to Sealing. Press the Pressure Cook or Manual button and set the cook time to 20 minutes.

When the Instant Pot beeps, allow the pressure to release naturally for 10 minutes, then carefully switch the Pressure Release valve to Venting. When fully released, open the lid. Carefully remove the muffins.

Nutrition Facts

Calories 71, Total Fat 4.8g, Saturated Fat 3.6g, Cholesterol 41mg, Sodium 248mg, Total Carbohydrate

5.7g, Dietary Fiber 0.9g , Total Sugars 4g, Protein 1.9g

Strawberry Corn Muffins

Prep time: 15 min Cooking Time: 30 min serve: 2

Ingredients

½ cup chia seed flour

1/8 cup yellow cornmeal

½ tablespoon honey

1/8 teaspoon salt

1/8 teaspoons baking powder

1/8 teaspoon baking soda

¼ tablespoon olive oil

½ teaspoon vanilla extract

1 egg

½ cup buttermilk

¼ cup fresh strawberries

1 cup water

Instructions

In a large bowl, combine chia seed flour, cornmeal, honey, salt, baking powder and baking soda. In a separate bowl, beat together olive oil, vanilla and egg.

Stir egg mixture into dry ingredients alternating with the buttermilk just until moistened.

Gently fold in the Strawberries. Spoon batter into prepared muffin tins. Pour 1 cup water into the Instant Pot. Place the trivet inside. Place the muffin cups on the rack or pan.

Secure the lid and set the Pressure Release valve to Sealing. Press the Pressure Cook or Manual button and set the cook time to 20 minutes.

When the Instant Pot beeps, allow the pressure to release naturally for 10 minutes, then carefully switch the Pressure Release valve to Venting. When fully released, open the lid. Carefully remove the muffins.

Nutrition Facts

Calories 80, Total Fat 2.9g , Saturated Fat 0.8g, Cholesterol 42mg, Sodium 194mg, Total Carbohydrate

10.6g, Dietary Fiber 0.8g , Total Sugars 4.8g, Protein 3.2g

Raspberry Crumble Bars

Raspberry Crumble Bars are easy, healthy, keto, low-carb, paleo, and vegan breakfast bars. A delicious gluten-free dessert with only 7 grams of net carbs per slice.

Prep Time: 20 mins Cook Time: 30 mins Total Time: 50 mins

Ingredients

BOTTOM LAYER

2 cups Almond Flour

2 cups unsweetened desiccated coconut 1/2 cup Coconut Flour

4 tablespoons Coconut oil melted

6 tablespoons sugar free syrup or honey or maple syrup 2 tablespoons Vanilla extract

1/4 teaspoon salt

8-10 tablespoons Water

TOP LAYER

1cups Frozen Raspberries 1/4 cup Water

1/2 cup Chia seeds

1/4 cup sugar free syrup or maple syrup or honey 1 teaspoon Vanilla extract

1 cup Coconut chips 1/3 cup Almond Flour

1/2 cup unsweetened desiccated coconut

3 tablespoons sugar free natural li□uid sweetener or honey or maple syrup

2 tablespoons Coconut oil 1/4 teaspoon salt

Instructions

Preheat oven to 350°F (180°C).

Prepare an 8-inch square baking tray covered with parchment paper. Set aside.

BOTTOM LAYER

In a food processor with the S blade attachment, add the almond meal, desiccated coconut, coconut flour, honey, salt, coconut oil and vanilla, and water (start with 8 tbsp). Process until it gets crumbly and all the ingredients are coming together. If too crumbly - it means it does not form a dough ball when firmly pressed within your hands - add 2 extra tablespoons of water. I added 10 tablespoons of water. Always add 2 tbsp at a time and check with a small portion of the dough. If it holds well together, you added enough water.

Evenly press the batter into the prepared baking tray. I used my fingers and flattened the layer pressing with a spatula.

Using a fork, prick the base a few times on a few areas to prevent the base from popping when baking.

Bake for 15 minutes. Cooldown fully in the tray before spreading the raspberry jam on top.

RASPBERRY CHIA SEED JAM

While the bottom layer is baking, prepare the jam. In a small saucepan, add all the jam ingredients. Cook the jam under medium heat, constantly stirring to avoid burning the jam. It is ready when the raspberries are fully melted, and it forms a thick jam. It should not take more than 5-6 minutes.

Set aside in a bowl to fully cool down and thicken a little bit. You can bring the jam outside on the deck to cool down faster. It does not have to be cold, room temperature is fine.

Spread the jam onto the baked bottom layer and return in the oven for 10 minutes to set. Remove from the oven. Set aside while you prepare the top layer.

TOP LAYER

Add all the top layer ingredients into a mixing bowl. Use your hand to combine the ingredients, rubbing the coconut oil and liquid sweetener onto the dry ingredients to create a crumbly batter. It is the messy part!

Crumble these ingredients on top of the last layer - the chia jam

- and return the tray to the oven for 10 minutes to slightly toast the coconut crumble layer.

Fully cool down for 1 hour in the pan. You can place the pan in a cooler place like outside on the deck to cool down faster. The jam must be set and at room temperature before making slices. Place the pan for 1 hour in the fridge to set the jam faster and make it easier to slice.

This recipe makes 16 slices. Store up to 1 week in the pantry in an airtight plastic box.

Nutrition Info

Calories 253

Calories from Fat 216 Fat 24g37% Carbohydrates 21.8g Fiber 14g58% Sugar 5.3g6% Protein 4.5g

Keto almond flour chocolate chip cookies

Prep Time: 10 mins Cook Time: 12 mins Total Time: 22 mins

Ingredients

5.3 oz Unsalted Butter soft, roughly diced, at room temperature for 3 hours

1/2 cup Erythritol

1/4 cup Golden erythritol or more erythritol 1 large Egg at room temperature

1 teaspoon Vanilla extract

1/2 teaspoon Almond extract optional but tasty! 1/4 teaspoon Salt

1/2 teaspoon Baking soda

1/4 teaspoon Xanthan gum highly recommended, add chewy texture, avoid cookies to crumble

2 1/4 cup Almond Flour

3/4 cup Sugar-free Chocolate Chips

Instructions

Preheat oven to 180°C (375°F). Line two cookie sheets with parchment paper. Set aside.

In a large mixing bowl, beat the soft butter with erythritol and golden erythritol until light and fluffy. It should take about 45 seconds on medium speed.

Stop the beater then add in egg, vanilla, almond extract, salt, baking soda and xanthan gum. I highly recommend xanthan gum as this adds a chewy texture to your cookies and it prevent the cookies to crumble easily.

Beat again on low speed until creamy.

Beat in the almond flour on medium speed, adding the flour 1/2 cup at a time. The batter will be fluffy and more difficult to beat as it goes, that is what you want.

Stop the beater and stir in the chocolate chips with a spatula.

Storage

Refrigerate the dough for 5 minutes.

Scoop out 3 tablespoons of dough per cookie and transfer onto a baking tray, covered with a piece of parchment paper. Leave 2 thumbs space between each cookie as they will expand during baking.

Depending on the texture and shape you aim to, slightly flatten each cookie ball into a disc. For a ultra thin, wide, cookie, flat in the center, press the cookie up to 4 mm (0.2 inches). For a thicker, softer/fluffier cookie give a small pression and barely flatten the dough. Remember that the thinner the crispier they will be in the center.

Bake 10-12 minutes, in center rack, until golden on the side but still white and soft in the middle.

Remove rack from the oven and cool the cookies on the rack for 12 minutes. Don't touch them at this point, they can be fragile and crumbly.

After 12 minutes, slide a spatula under each cookies to transfer them to a cooling rack.

Cool 20 more minutes on the cooling rack before eating. Note that the cookies will get their final texture only after 4 hours on the cooling rack at room temperature. For a crispier cookie, store in the fridge! Serve with a pinch of salt to enhance the flavors.

Nutrition Info

Calories 201 Calories from Fat 162 Fat 18g

Saturated Fat 7g Cholesterol 32mg Sodium 143mg Potassium 7mg Carbohydrates 5g Fiber 2g

Sugar 1g Protein 4g

Vegan Chocolate Peanut Butter Cookies

Vegan Chocolate Peanut Butter Cookies are healthy coconut flour vegan cookies with a shortbread crunchy and sandy texture made with only 4 ingredients.

Prep Time: 10 mins Cook Time: 12 mins Total Time: 22 mins

Ingredients

1 cup Natural Peanut butter fresh, runny 1/4 cup Coconut Flour sifted, no lumps

2 tablespoons unsweetened cocoa powder

1/4 cup sugar-free natural liquid sweetener or maple syrup

Instructions

Preheat oven to 180C (356F).

Prepare a cookie rack covered with parchment paper. Set aside. In a food processor with the S blade attachment, add all the ingredients, order doesn't matter. Process on medium speed for about 1 minute or until all the ingredients come together into a ball.

Stop the food processor, gather the ingredients together to form a ball and split in 8 even pieces.

Roll each piece into a cookie ball, place each ball on the prepared cookie rack leaving half thumb space between each cookies. The cookies won't spread so you don't have to leave too much space. If the dough is too dry or crumbly, you can oil your hands with a tiny amount of coconut oil to make the rolling easier.

Bake for 10-12 minutes.

Cool down on a cookie rack. I used a large spatula that I slide under the cookie to gently transfer the cookies one by one to the rack without breaking them.

When cool down, decorate with sugar free melted dark chocolate and chop peanuts. Place the cookies in the freezer for a few minutes to □uickly set the melted chocolate if needed.

Store up to 3 weeks in a cookie jar.

Nutrition Info

Calories 218 Calories from Fat 140 Fat 15.6g24%

Saturated Fat 2.4g Carbohydrates 10.6g Fiber 5.2g22% Sugar 2.6g3% Protein 9.3g

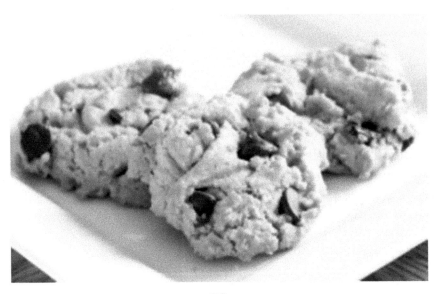

Keto Gingerbread cookies vegan and gluten-free

Keto Gingerbread cookies an easy healthy gluten-free cookie recipe without molasses. A delicious crispy Christmas cookie for kids or cookie lovers.

Prep Time: 10 mins Cook Time: 20 mins Total Time: 50 mins

Ingredients

Dry ingredients

2 cup Almond Flour or almond meal 1/2 cup Erythritol or golden monk fruit 1 teaspoon Ground ginger

1/2 tablespoon Ground cinnamon

1 teaspoon Baking Powder or 1/2 teaspoon baking soda 1/4 teaspoon ground cloves

Wet ingredients

1 large Egg or 1 tablespoon chia seed + 3 tablespoons water 1/4 cup Coconut oil melted or butter

1 teaspoon Vanilla extract

1 tablespoon black strap molasse - optional, recipe work without it but great iron boost for vegan

Keto royal icing

1 cup sugar free icing sugar

1-2 tablespoon Unsweetened Almond Milk 1/4 teaspoon guar gum

Instructions

Preheat oven to 180°C (350°F) and line two cookie baking sheets with parchment paper. Set aside.

If you are vegan and don't want to use an egg, add chia seed and water in a small bowl. Stir. Set aside 10 minutes until it forms a gel.

In a large mixing bowl, combine the dry ingredients: almond flour, erythritol, and spices.

Add the beaten egg (or chia seed gel if keto vegan), melted coconut oil, molasses (optional!), and vanilla extract.

Combine with a spatula first, then use your hands and knead the dough until it comes together.

Divide the dough into two balls of the same size. Wrap each ball tightly into plastic wrap, roughly flatten into a thick disc and refrigerate both discs for 1 hour.

Remove the dough discs from the fridge, unwrap one disc and place it in the center of two parchment paper pieces.

Roll out the dough into a 1/2 inch thickness (for thicker cookies) or 1/4 inch thick (for thinner cookies).

Use a gingerbread man cookie cutter shape to cut out cookies - I made 6 cookies in each half-disc of dough, so 12 in total. My tip: use a small knife or spatula to lift the shaped cookie and transfer it onto the prepared baking cookie sheets.

Gather up the leftover dough into a ball and re-roll to form more cookies. You should be able to shape 12 large gingerbread cookies with the entire recipe, depending on your cookie cutter size.

Bake your cookies for 12-14 minutes max or until the border are golden brown.

Remove from the oven, cool down 5 minutes on the baking sheet, then gently transfer into a cooling rack. I recommend using a spatula that you slide under each cookie to transfer them gently. They will look soft, and that is ok! They will firm up with time. Cool them down for at least 20 minutes. Be patient; the cookies will get very crunchy with time! Trust me, after a few hours. You won't believe how crunchy and flavorsome they get! The gingerbread flavor will also enhance after 24 hours.

Store up to 2 weeks in a cookie jar, in the pantry.

Keto royal icing

Combine sugar-free icing powder with almond milk and guar gum until it forms a white paste.

Use a piping bag to pipe shapes on the cookies.

Dry at room temperature. It can take up to 48 hours for the decorations to harden.

Nutrition Info

Calories 138

Calories from Fat 100 Fat 11.1g Carbohydrates 5.1g Fiber 2.6g Protein 4.2g

Keto no-bake cookies

Keto no-bake cookies are low carb peanut butter chocolate cookies packed with healthy coconut oil, flaxseed meal, and walnuts.

Prep Time: 10 mins Total Time: 30 mins

Ingredients

Dry ingredients

1 cup Almond Flour

1 cup unsweetened desiccated coconut 1 cup Walnuts , roughly chopped

2 1/2 tablespoons unsweetened cocoa powder 2 tablespoons Flaxseed meal

1/3 cup Erythritol or if paleo (not sugar free) you can use coconut sugar

Wet ingredients

3/4 cup Natural Peanut butter or nut butter you like 1/4 cup + 2 tablespoons Coconut oil

1 teaspoon Vanilla essence Chocolate glazing

1/2 cup Sugar-free Chocolate Chips or stevia sweetened chocolate

1/3 cup Coconut cream - thick part from top of can

2-4 drops stevia li☐uid optional, adjust regarding desired sweetness

Instructions

Line parchment paper on one or two plates. Make sure the plates fit in your freezer as you must freeze these cookies to set.

You may need more plates depending on your plate size. Set aside.

In a large mixing bowl, add all the dry ingredients EXCEPT the sugar-free sweetener (erythritol).

Stir to combine. Set aside.

In another mixing bowl, add peanut butter, coconut oil, vanilla, and erythritol. Microwave by 30 seconds bursts, stirring in between. Repeat until the coconut oil is fully melted and all the ingredients are combined. It should not take more than 1 minute 30 seconds.

If you don't have a microwave available, bring the ingredients into a small saucepan, warm under medium heat, stirring all the time until it forms a consistent mixture.

Stir in the peanut butter mixture onto the dry ingredients. Make sure the liquid covers all the dry ingredients, the batter will be quite wet and that's what you want.

Scoop out some cookie dough onto the prepared plate covered with parchment paper. You should be able to divide the batter into 12 large cookies.

Spread the dough with the back of a spoon to form a cookie shape.

Freeze for 20 minutes, until the cookies are hard. Meanwhile, prepare the chocolate glazing.

Chocolate glazing

In a mixing bowl add the sugar-free chocolate chips, coconut cream, and stevia drops. Microwave by 30 seconds bursts as you did before until the chocolate is fully melted. It will create a slightly thick chocolate cream.

Remove the cookies from the freezer.

Scoop out some of the chocolate glazing in the middle of each cookie and spread with the back of the spoon. Repeat for each cookie, until no more glazing left.

Decorate each no-bake keto cookie by adding walnuts halves in the center.

Return to the freezer 2-3 minutes to set the glazing. Enjoy your no-bake cookies!

This recipe makes about 12 large no-bake cookies.

Storage: They must be stored in an airtight container in the fridge or they will soften even melt during summer. Store up to 3-4 weeks in the fridge. You can also freeze these cookies and defrost 1 hour before eating.

Nutrition Info

Calories 194 Calories from Fat 152 Fat 16.9g26%

Carbohydrates 8.2g Fiber 3.3g14% Sugar 3.6g4% Protein 4.9g

Coconut flour cookies no sugar

Don't blow your diet this Christmas! Whatever you eat keto, low carb, paleo or vegan, these coconut flour cookies have no sugar. It's the healthy Christmas cookies you need to make everyone happy.

Prep Time: 15 mins Cook Time: 8 mins Total Time: 23 mins 12 cookies

Ingredients

Decoration

3/4 cup Coconut Flour

1/3 cup Coconut oil solid, not melted +/- 1 tablespoon (add if the dough is too crumbly)

1/4 cup Erythritol - monk fruit sugar or erythritol 1/4 teaspoon Vanilla extract

1 large Egg - at room temperature, or 1 tablespoon of peanut butter if vegan keto

1/3 cup Sugar-free Dark Chocolate I used stevia chocolate 1 tablespoon Pumpkin seeds crushed

1 teaspoon unsweetened desiccated coconut Optional - to sprinkle on top before baking

1 tablespoon Coconut Flour

Instructions

Preheat oven to fan-bake 180°C (350°F). Prepare a cookie tray, cover with parchment paper. Set aside.

Place all the ingredients in a bowl, beat with an electric beater until it forms a crumble. It should not take more than 20 seconds. If you don't have an electric beater you can also press/rub the dough with your hands until it forms a crumb - just a bit messier!

Assemble the crumb with your hands to form a cookie dough ball and transfer the ball onto a piece of plastic wrap. It's a crumbly dough, that's normal, press firmly with your hands to gather the pieces together and firmly wrap the batter to form a ball. If it really doesn't come together after you kneaded the dough for 1 minute, add slightly more coconut oil - up to 1 tablespoon max. Refrigerate for 15 minutes to firm up.

Remove from the fridge, open the plastic wrap, the dough will be firm but still crumbly when you take some in your hands that is ok. The more you knead the dough the easier it gets to form balls as the coconut oil softens.

Roll 1 tablespoon of dough into a ball, pressing the dough firmly in your hands. Place the balls onto the prepared baking sheet. If you want to make crescent-shaped cookies. First, shape the ball into a cylinder, slightly pinch the middle to form a crescent shape. The fastest will be to simply flatten the ball with a fork to form lovely round shortbread cookies. Repeat with remaining dough until you form 12 cookies.

If you like, sprinkle extra coconut flour on top of the cookies before baking.

Bake until light golden brown on the sides 6 to 8 minutes. The cookies will remain very soft at this stage and that is normal, don't touch them or don't try to remove them from the tray, they firm up when fully cool down.

Cool down on the baking sheet for about 30 minutes until it reaches room temperature. As it cools down, the coconut oil hardens and creates crispy crumbly shortbread cookies. I usually place my baking sheet outside in summer to cool down in fresh air quickly or near an open window.

Decorate with a drizzle of melted sugar-free chocolate if you like. I used dark chocolate sweetened with stevia.

Nutrition Info

Calories 208 Calories from Fat 175 Fat 19.4g Carbohydrates 6g Fiber 3.3g Sugar 2g2% Protein 2.5g

Low carb lemon cookies

Low carb lemon cookies are easy, healthy soft buttery cookies, with no butter and a bursting lemon juice flavor. 100 % Vegan + Keto + Gluten free these healthy lemon cookies with almond flour suit all diet.

Prep Time: 10 mins Cook Time: 15 mins Total Time: 55 mins

Ingredients

Dry ingredients

1 1/3 cup Almond Flour

2 tablespoons Coconut Flour

1/4 cup Erythritol - can go up to 1/3 cup for a sweeter flavor 1/2 teaspoon Baking soda

Li□uid ingredients

1/4 cup Lemon Juice fresh or organic 1/4 cup Coconut oil

1 tablespoon Lemon Zest - optional Sugar-free lemon glazing

1/4 cup Sugar-free powdered sweetener 2 teaspoons Lemon Juice

1 teaspoon Coconut oil , melted

1 tablespoon Lemon Zest , optional, to decorate

Instructions

Preheat oven to 180°C (350°F). Line a cookie tray with parchment paper. Set aside.

In a medium mixing bowl, combine all the dry ingredients: almond flour, coconut flour, sugar-free crystal sweetener and baking soda. Set aside.

In a small mixing bowl, add coconut oil and lemon juice. Microwave for 30 seconds, stir and repeat until the coconut oil is fully melted. Otherwise, place the ingredients in a saucepan warm on medium heat. Remove from heat when the coconut oil is melted.

Pour li☐uid onto dry ingredients, add lemon zest if desired, and combine until it forms a cookie dough. You should be able to shape a ball. The batter should be soft, buttery, and not dry. If dry, adjust with 1-2 teaspoon of water but you shouldn't have to.

Refrigerate for 10 minutes, wrapped in a piece of plastic wrap or in the mixing bowl covered with silicone lid.

Remove the dough from the fridge and shape 8 even cookie dough balls. You can weigh the dough if you want precision.

Roll each ball in your hands to shape smooth cookie dough balls.

Place each ball on the cookie tray leaving a thumb-size space between each ball. The cookies won't expand in the oven so you don't have to leave a big space between them.

Press the balls slightly with your hand palm to flatten cookies. Don't flatten too much or the sides will form cracks and they won't be as soft and moist. The thicker, the moister!

Bake for 15 minutes or until golden on sides. The middle will stay slightly soft and that is the texture you want.

Remove the cookie tray from the oven and cool down on the tray for 20 minutes before transferring on the rack to cool down to room temperature. Don't touch the cookies during the first 20 minutes, they are soft and need time to firm up.

Prepare the sugar-free lemon glazing

In a small mixing bowl, combine the sugar-free powdered sweetener, coconut oil, and lemon juice. Play with the texture, adding more sweetener, 1 teaspoon at a time for a thicker glazing or more lemon juice for a thinner glazing.

Drizzle the glazing onto the cold cookies. Don't decorate warm or lukewarm cookies or the glazing will melt and be absorbed by the cookie dough.

For a lovely, white glazing, place the cookies 2 minutes in the

freezer just after adding the glazing. This step sets the glazing fast and makes beautiful cookie decorations.

Sprinkle lemon zest on top if desired.

Store the lemon cookies in an airtight container for up to 3 days in the pantry or in the fridge if you prefer your cookies firm.

Nutrition Info

Calories 194 Calories from Fat 102 Fat 11.3g17% Carbohydrates 6.6g2% Fiber 2.4g10% Protein 3.4g

Almond Flour Chocolate Chip Cookies

These Vegan Almond Flour Chocolate Chip Cookies are Paleo, Low-Carb, Sugar-free, easy 6-ingredient healthy cookies with only 5.8g net carbs per cookie.

Prep Time: 10 mins Cook Time: 12 mins Total Time: 22 mins

Ingredients

2 cups Almond Flour also known as almond flour or ground almond

1/4 cup Coconut oil melted

1/4 cup Sugar-free flavored maple syrup or li□uid sweetener of choice (maple syrup if paleo or vegan)

1/4 teaspoon Salt + extra to sprinkle on top (optional) 1/2 teaspoon Baking soda

1/3 cup Sugar-free Chocolate Chips or >85% cocoa 2 teaspoons Vanilla extract

Instructions

Preheat oven to 180°C (350°F).

Line a cookie sheet with parchment paper. Set aside.

In a large mixing bowl add almond meal, li□uid sweetener, melted coconut oil, vanilla, salt, and baking soda.

Combine with a spatula or a spoon until all the ingredients are combined and it forms pieces/crumble of cookie dough.

Use your hands to bring the pieces together into a large cookie dough ball. The dough is soft, easy to bring together into a ball, not a crumbly dough.

Roll the dough ball into a cylinder of about 20 cm long (7 inches long), use a sharp knife to divide the cylinder into 8 even pieces. I usually make 8 medium size cookies but feel free to make 6 large cookies if preferred!

Take a piece of dough, roll into a ball and place the cookie dough ball on the cookie sheet. Repeat for the other pieces of dough. Leave about a thumb space between each cookie dough ball – the cookies won't expand much when baking so you don't need lots of space between balls. Repeat for all cookie balls until you obtain 8 cookie balls on the cookie sheet covered with parchment paper.

Flatten each cookie ball with your hands. The more you press the thinner and crispier they will be. Don't press too much for a softer, chewier, and thicker cookie. If the border slightly cracks, simply use your finger to smooth the border and reshape.

Add a few dark chocolate chunks or chips onto each flattened cookies. Slightly press to stick the chocolate to the dough- not much as you don't want the chips/chunks to go through the dough. Place the chocolate chunks away from the border, to prevent the chocolate from overflowing from the cookie when baking.

Bake 12 minutes or until the edges are golden.

They will be slightly soft when out of the oven, cool down 5 minutes on the baking sheet then using a spatula, transfer onto a cooling rack.

Store for 1 week in a cookie jar.

Nutrition Info

Calories 234 Calories from Fat 172 Fat 19.1g Carbohydrates 11.2g Fiber 5.4g% Sugar 1.1g1% Protein 6.2g

Keto Coconut cookies

Prep Time: 10 mins Cook Time: 15 mins Total Time: 25 mins

Ingredients

2 cup unsweetened desiccated coconut 200g 1 1/2 cup Almond Flour 160g

2 large Egg or 2 flax eggs if vegan 1/2 cup Coconut oil melted, or butter 1/2 cup Erythritol (100g)

1 teaspoon Vanilla essence Cookies decoration

1 teaspoons unsweetened desiccated coconut toasted if desired

Instructions

Preheat oven to 180°C (360°F). Lay a cookie sheet with baking paper. Set aside.

In a food processor, with the S blade attachment, add all the cookie ingredients.

Process on medium speed until all the ingredients come together. Scoop out the dough with a cookie scoop, and roll into a ball with your hands

Place each cookie ball on the baking tray covered with baking paper. You should be able to make 10 large cookies with the whole batter.

Press each ball with your fingers to form thick flat round cookies - about 1 cm thickness.

Bake at 180°C (360°F) for 18-23 minutes or until the sides and top are golden-brown.

Cool down on the cookie sheet for 20 minutes, they will harden slightly when cooling down.

Storage

Transfer onto a cookie rack to fully cool down to room temperature.

Store up to 5 days in a cookie jar or freeze for later.

Nutrition Info

Calories 190 Calories from Fat 107 Fat 11.9g Carbohydrates 6.3g Fiber 2.2g Sugar 1.4g Protein 4.5g

Cookie dough bars no bake, keto, vegan

Cookie Dough Bars are delicious no-bake peanut butter chocolate chips bars made with only 5 wholesome ingredients. A healthy 100% keto, low-carb, sugar-free, gluten-free, and vegan bar ready in only 30 minutes to fix a sweet craving with no guilt.

Prep Time: 10 mins Total Time: 30 mins

Ingredients

3/4 cup Almond Flour or almond flour 2 tablespoons Coconut Flour

1/2 cup Natural Peanut butter unsalted, fresh, runny 2 tablespoons Sugar-free flavored maple syrup

1/3 cup Sugar-free Chocolate Chips Chocolate nut butter layer

3 oz Sugar-free Dark Chocolate

2 tablespoons Natural Peanut butter unsalted, fresh, runny

Instructions

In a medium bowl combine the liquid sweetener and peanut butter.

Microwave 30 seconds - it will be slightly warm, stir to combine. Set aside.

Add the almond flour, coconut flour, and chocolate chips.

Stir until fully incorporated. It will form a dough that you can easily shape as a cookie dough ball.

Transfer the dough into a rectangle loaf baking pan covered with a piece of parchment paper. (my loaf pan is a 9-inch x 5- inch x 1.8-inch pan)

Press the dough with your hands to cover all the bottom of the pan. Use a spatula to make the surface flat and smooth. Freeze while you prepare the chocolate layer.

In a bowl combine the sugar-free dark chocolate and nut butter. Melt by 30 seconds bursts in the microwave stirring between to prevent the chocolate from burning. It should not re□uire more than 90 seconds. Stir well to combine and form a shiny melted chocolate mixture.

Remove the loaf pan from the freezer, pour the melted chocolate onto the bar. Use a spatula to spread the layer evenly. Freeze again for 10-15 minutes or until the chocolate layer is set.

Cut into bars using a sharp knife. You can warm the knife blade slightly to make the cutting even easier. This recipe makes 8 square bars.

Store the bars in the fridge in an airtight plastic container or plastic bag for up to 10 days!

Nutrition Info

Calories 198 Calories from Fat 149 Fat 16.5g25% Carbohydrates 9.9g Fiber 3.9g Sugar 3g3% Protein 7.2g

Paleo Pumpkin Brownies

Prep Time: 10 mins Cook Time: 25 mins Total Time: 55 mins 16 brownie squares

Ingredients

Paleo Pumpkin Brownies

1 cup Pumpkin Puree , canned, no sugar added

1 cup almond butter , smooth, fresh, no added sugar, no added oil (or use peanut butter)

1/2 cup Sugar-free flavored maple syrup or maple syrup (if not sugar free)

1 teaspon Vanilla extract

1 teaspoon pumpkin pie spices

1 cup unsweetened cocoa powder

1/3 cup Sugar-free Chocolate Chips or dark chocolate chips 85% cocoa

Pumpkin glazing

1/3 cup almond butter , smooth, fresh, no added sugar, no added oil (or use peanut butter)

1 tablespoon Coconut oil , melted

1 tablespoon Pumpkin Puree ,canned, no sugar added 1/4 teaspoon pumpkin pie spices

1-2 Monk Fruit Drops or Stevia Drops - optional Chocolate drizzle

2 oz Sugar-free Chocolate Chips or dark chocolate 85% cocoa 1/2 teaspoon Coconut oil

Instructions

Preheat oven to 180C (350F).

Line a s□uare brownie pan with parchment paper. Set aside.

In a food processor, using the S blade attachment add the pumpkin puree, almond butter, sugar free maple flavored syrup, pumpkin spices and vanilla.

Blend on high speed for 30 seconds or until it forms a consistent batter with a lovely orange color.

Add unsweetened cocoa powder and blend again for 30 seconds until it forms a thick, sticky and shiny brownie batter.

Stir in the chocolate chips using a spatula or the pulse mode of your food processor.

Transfer the brownie batter into the prepared brownie pan and spread evenly using a silicone spatula. The batter is sticky and that is what you want.

Sprinkle extra sugar free chocolate chips on top. Lightly press them into the batter using the spatula.

Bake for 20-25 minutes or until the top and edge are set. Remove from the oven, let cool down 15 minutes into the brownie pan.

Transfer onto a cooling rack. Meanwhile prepare the pumpkin glaze.

Pumpkin glaze

In a medium mixing bowl, add nut butter, melted coconut oil, pumpkin spices, pumpkin puree and pumpkin stevia drops.

Combine with a spoon until it forms a creamy glazing.

Drizzle on top of the cool brownie until no more left. The glazing won't harden it will stay moist and soft.

Chocolate drizzle - optional

In a microwave safe bowl, melt the sugar free chocolate chips with melted coconut oil. Microwave by 30 seconds burst, stir and repeat until fully melted. Drizzle on top of the pumpkin glazing.

You can freeze the brownie 10 minutes to set the chocolate drizzle and add an extra fudgy texture to the brownie.

Store the brownie for up to 4 days in the fridge using a cake box to prevent the brownie to dry. You can also store at room temperature up to 2 days.

Brownie can be freeze in zip bags.

Nutrition Info

Calories 154.5 Calories from Fat 120 Fat 13.3g20% Saturated Fat 2.2g Sodium 3.4mg0% Potassium 269.3mg8% Carbohydrates 8.4g3% Fiber 4.4g18% Sugar 1.6g2% Protein 5.6g

No bake peanut butter bars healthy

No bake peanut butter bars healthy dessert made with 6 simple ingredients, 100% sugar-free, gluten-free and vegan. A delicious easy low-carb recipe to fix your sweet cravings with no sugar in less than 20 minutes.

Prep Time: 15 mins Total Time: 35 mins 12 bars

Ingredients

Peanut butter layer

1 cup Natural Peanut butter unsalted, no oil added (265g) 2/3 cup Coconut Flour (72g)

1/3 cup Sugar-free powdered sweetener or powdered monk fruit/stevia blend (53g)

Chocolate Peanut butter layer

1/3 cup unsweetened cocoa powder

2 tablepoon Natural Peanut butter unsalted, no added oil or sugar (30ml)

4 tablespoon Coconut oil , melted (60ml)

2 tablespoon Sugar-free powdered sweetener

Instructions

In a medium mixing bowl, add peanut butter, coconut flour and powdered sugar-free sweetener of your choice.

Combine with a spatula, then knead with your hand to form a consistent peanut butter dough.

Transfer the peanut butter dough into a rectangle loaf baking pan covered with a piece of parchment paper. I used a cake loaf pan size: 9 inches x 5 inches X 1.8 inches.

Press the dough to cover the bottom of the pan evenly. Use a spatula to smooth the top.

Put the pan in the freezer while you prepare the chocolate peanut butter layer.

In a small mixing bowl add peanut butter and coconut oil. Microwave 30 seconds, or bring on the stove for 1 minute under low heat, stirring constantly to combine both ingredients. Stir in powdered sugar-free sweetener and unsweetened cocoa powder. Make sure you stir the mixture fast to avoid any lumps or otherwise gradually add the powdered ingredients stirring after each addition.

Remove the loaf pan from the freezer. Spread the chocolate layer on top of the peanut butter layer. It should set really fast as your base is very cold. Spread evenly using a spatula.

Freeze 30 minutes before slicing into 12 slices. Warm the knife blade under heat before cutting, it prevents the chocolate layer from breaking.

Storage

These bars are soft and must be stored in an airtight container in the fridge. Can store up to 4 weeks or freeze and eat frozen or defrost 30 minutes-1 hour before eating.

Nutrition Info

Calories 215 Calories from Fat 162 Fat 18g Carbohydrates 10.7g Fiber 4g Protein 7.8g

Chocolate-chip cookie ice-cream sandwiches

Prep:20 mins Cook:20 mins   Plus overnight chilling Easy
Makes 12 sandwiches or 24 cookies

Ingredients

280g brown sugar

225g sugar

250g butter

2 large eggs

1 tbsp vanilla extract

450g plain flour

2 tsp baking powder

300g milk chocolate

vanilla ice cream

Directions:

To make the cookies, tip the sugars and butter into a large bowl. Get a grown-up to help you use an electric hand mixer to blend them until the mixture looks smooth and creamy, and a little paler in colour.

Carefully break in the eggs, one at a time, mixing well between each egg and pausing to scrape down the sides with a spatula. Mix in the vanilla.

Sift in the flour and baking powder, then mix well with a wooden spoon.Stir through the chocolate chunks. Use your hands to squeeze the dough together in 1 big lump, split into 2 even pieces. Put each piece on a sheet of cling film.

Roll each piece of dough in the cling film to form thick sausage shapes and then seal the ends. Put them in the fridge and chill for at least 3 hrs or overnight – can be frozen at this point.

Heat oven to 180C/160C fan/ gas 4. Take the dough rolls out of the fridge, unwrap and use a small knife to slice each one into 12 pieces, so you have 24 in total.

Place the slices on a baking tray lined with baking parchment. Put this in the oven to bake for 20 mins or until the cookies are golden brown on the edges, but still pale in the centre.

Allow to cool slightly before lifting them onto a wire rack to cool completely. Sandwich the cookies together with ice cream and dig in!

Keto Granola Bars

Easy chewy no-bake hemp seeds bars 100% Nut-Free, Grain-Free, and Vegan with only 4.2 grams of net carbs and 9 grams of protein per bar.

Prep Time: 25 mins Total Time: 25 mins 10 granola bars

Ingredients

Dry ingredients

1/2 cup Sunflower seed butter

3 tablespoons Coconut oil

1/4 cup Sugar-free flavored maple syrup

1 teaspoon Vanilla extract

1 cup hemp hearts - raw, shelled also known as hemp seeds

1 tablespoon Chia seeds

1/3 cup Pumpkin seeds

1/4 cup Sunflower seeds

1/3 cup Coconut chips

1/2 teaspoon Cinnamon

2 tablespoons Erythritol - or /3 stevia drops (optional, to adjust sweetness)

Chocolate drizzle

1/4 cup Sugar-free Chocolate Chips 1 teaspoon Coconut oil

Instructions

Line a 9-inch x 5-inch loaf pan with parchment paper. Set aside.

In a medium mixing bowl, add all the dry ingredients, the order doesn't matter. Stir, set aside.

In another mixing bowl, add sunflower seed butter, melted coconut oil, sugar-free syrup, and vanilla.

Microwave 30 seconds, stir, microwave 30 seconds again if your sunflower seed butter is too hard to combine. You must obtain a thick brownish paste. If you don't have a microwave, bring on a stove in a small saucepan, stirring often until the ingredients are combined.

Pour the seed butter mixture onto the dry ingredients and combine with a spoon until the mixture covers all the dry ingredients evenly.

Transfer the mixture into the prepared loaf pan, press with a spatula firmly to compact the granola bar mixture as much as you can.

Freeze 20 minutes to set.

Chocolate drizzle

Meanwhile, melt the sugar-free chocolate chips and coconut oil in a small bowl. You can microwave by 30 seconds burst, or use a saucepan under medium heat.

Bring the bar out of the freezer. Lift the parchment paper to pull out the bar from the loaf pan and place it on a plate or chopping board.

Drizzle the melted chocolate on top of the bar and bring the bar back to the freezer for 2 minutes to set the chocolate.

Cut into 10 bars, I recommend you warm the knife blade under a flame or hot water (dry the blade to avoid water to be added to the bar).

Storage and freezing

Store the bars in the fridge in an airtight container for up to 3 weeks or wrap individually into plastic wrap and freeze up to 3 months.

These bars must be kept in the fridge as they soften after 20 minutes out of the fridge.

Nutrition Info

Calories 285 Calories from Fat 224 Fat 24.9g38% Carbohydrates 13.5g Fiber 9.2g38% Protein 9.2g

Keto Strawberry Pop Tarts

A buttery flaky pastry filled with sugar-free chia seed jam Prep Time: 15 mins

Cook Time: 20 mins Total Time: 35 mins 8 pop tarts

Ingredients

Keto pastry doughFilling

2 1/4 cup Almond Flour, fine, blanched (250g)

1/2 cup Coconut Flour fresh, no lump, packed, leveled up (60g)

1/4 cup Erythritol - erythritol (swerve) or Monk fruit (Lakanto)

2 1/2 teaspoon Xanthan gum - don't skip!

1/3 cup + 1 tbsp Unsweetened Almond Milk

3.5 oz Melted Unsalted Butter (100g) or dairy-free vegan butter 1/2 tablespoon Apple cider vinegar

To decorate

6 tablespoons Sugar free chia seed jam

6 tablespons Cream Cheese or vegan coconut yoghurt

1/4 cup Sugar-free powdered sweetener

1/2-1 tablespoon Unsweetened Almond Milk adjust to taste

Instructions

Before you start, make sure you measure all the ingredients precisely either in grams/oz or cups. If you use cups firmly pack flours in the cup and level up.

Preheat oven to 180C (350F). Line a baking tray with parchment paper. Set aside.

In a large mixing bowl, whisk all the dry ingredients together : almond flour, coconut flour, sugar-free crystal sweetener and xanthan gum.

Add in unsweetened almond milk, melted butter, and apple cider vinegar.

Combine with a spoon at first then knead the dough with your hands until you are able to shape a ball.

Wrap the pastry dough ball into a piece of parchment paper or cling film wrap.

Freeze 10 minutes.

Remove the dough from the freezer and divide the dough ball in half. Roll each half between two pieces of parchment paper into a 1/4 inches thick rectangles about 1.5 x 2.3 inches (4cm x 6 cm). You will get around 16 small rectangles in total, 8 from each half dough balls. For larger tarts, double size of each rectangles and make only 6 pop tarts (net carb will conse□uently double up too)

Transfer rectangles of dough onto the prepared baking tray, leaving 1 thumb space between each rectangle. The dough won't expand while baking but the jam may run out the pastry so it's better to leave some space between each pop tart.

Spread 1/2 tablespoon of cream cheese (or vegan coconut yoghurt) in the center of each rectangle of dough leaving 1/2 inch (1 cm) border around the edges. Layer 1/2 tablespoon of chia seed jam on each rectangle over the cream cheese and add few slices of fresh strawberries (optional) . Make sure you don't cover the borders of the rectangle with the filling or you won't be able to close the tart. Use less filling if needed (this can happen if you roll your dough thicker and didn't manage to cut out enough rectangles)

Lay the other rectangles over the filling and seal the edges by pressing with your fingertips. If desired, cut the top dough with a knife to form gills - optional.

Brush the top of each pop tarts with beaten eggs or unsweetened almond milk if vegan.

Bake for 25 minutes in the center rack of your until the crust is golden brown. You can add a piece of foil on top of the pop tarts if the crust brown to dark/too fast and bring the tray to a level lower in the oven.

Meanwhile, in a small bowl combine sugar-free powdered sweetener with almond milk. Add more almond milk to make the glazing more li□uid or add more powdered sweetener to thicken.

Cool down the pop tarts on a rack for 2 hours. Drizzle the glazing onto the cold pop tarts

Store in an airtight container in the fridge for up to 3 days or freeze individually and defrost the day before at room temperature.

Nutrition Info

Calories 307 Calories from Fat 151 Fat 16.8g Carbohydrates 11g Fiber 4.4g18% Sugar 2.6g3% Protein 6.3g

Crispy chocolate fridge cake

Prep:20 mins Cook:5 mins Plus chilling Easy Makes 16-20 chunks

Ingredients

300g dark chocolate

100g butter 140g golden syrup 2 tsp vanilla extract

220g biscuit

120g sultana 85g Rice Krispies

140g mini eggs

50g white chocolate

Directions:

Line a 20 x 30cm tin with baking parchment. Melt the chocolate, butter and golden syrup in a bowl set over a pan of simmering water, stirring occasionally, until smooth and glossy. Add the vanilla, biscuits, sultanas and Rice Krispies, and mix well until everything is coated.

Tip the mixture into the tin, then flatten it down with the back of a spoon. Press in some mini eggs, if using, and put in the fridge until set. When hard, drizzle all over with the melted white chocolate and set again before cutting into chunks.

Oat Applesauce Muffins

Prep time: 15 min Cooking Time: 30 min serve: 2

Ingredients

¼ cup rolled oats

¼ cup buttermilk

¼ cup all-purpose flour

¼ teaspoon baking powder

¼ teaspoon baking soda

1/4 tablespoon honey

½ tablespoon applesauce

1 egg

1 cup water

Instructions

In a large bowl, stir together all-purpose flour, baking powder, baking soda and honey. Stir in oats and buttermilk mixture, applesauce and egg; mix well. Pour batter into prepared muffin cups.

Pour 1 cup water into the Instant Pot. Place the trivet inside. Place the muffin cups on the rack or pan.

Secure the lid and set the Pressure Release valve to Sealing. Press the Pressure Cook or Manual button and set the cook time to 20 minutes.

When the Instant Pot beeps, allow the pressure to release naturally for 10 minutes, then carefully switch the Pressure

Release valve to Venting. When fully released, open the lid. Carefully remove the muffins.

Nutrition Facts

Calories 150, Total Fat 3.3g, Saturated Fat 1g, Cholesterol 83mg, Sodium 223mg, Total Carbohydrate

Almond Banana Chocolate Muffins

Prep time: 15 min Cooking Time: 30 min serve: 2

Ingredients

1 banana

1 cup water

1 egg

¼ tablespoon coconut oil

¼ teaspoon applesauce

½ cup almond flour

1 tablespoon honey

¼ teaspoon baking powder

¼ teaspoon baking soda

½ cup sliced California almonds, divided

½ cup semi-sweet chocolate chips

Instructions

In a large bowl, stir together banana, almond flour, baking powder, baking soda and honey. Stir in coconut oil, applesauce and egg; chocolate chips and almond mix well. Pour batter into prepared muffin cups.

Pour 1 cup water into the Instant Pot. Place the trivet inside. Place the muffin cups on the rack or pan.

Press the Pressure Cook or Manual button and set the cook time to 20 minutes.

When the Instant Pot beeps, allow the pressure to release naturally for 10 minutes, then carefully switch the Pressure Release valve to Venting. When fully released, open the lid. Carefully remove the muffins.

Nutrition Facts

Calories 165, Total Fat 10.6g, Saturated Fat 2g Cholesterol 41mg , Sodium 29mg, Total Carbohydrate

12.3g, Dietary Fiber 2.8g , Total Sugars 5.7g, Protein 5.1g

Cinnamon Bran Muffins

Prep time: 15 min Cooking Time: 30 min serve: 2

Ingredients

1/2 cup bran flakes cereal

1 cup coconut flour

½ tablespoon honey

½ teaspoon baking powder

½ teaspoon ground cinnamon

½ cup buttermilk

1/2 tablespoon butter, melted

½ teaspoon vanilla extract

1 cup water

Instructions

In a large bowl, combine bran flakes, coconut flour, honey, baking powder and cinnamon. Stir in buttermilk, butter, and vanilla. Spoon mixture into prepared muffin cups.

Pour 1 cup water into the Instant Pot. Place the trivet inside. Place the muffin cups on the rack or pan.

Secure the lid and set the Pressure Release valve to Sealing. Press the Pressure Cook or Manual button and set the cook time to 20 minutes.

When the Instant Pot beeps, allow the pressure to release naturally for 10 minutes, then carefully switch the Pressure Release valve to Venting. When fully released, open the lid. Carefully remove the muffins.

Nutrition Facts

Calories 65, Total Fat 2.3g, Saturated Fat 1.6g, Cholesterol 5mg, Sodium 61mg, Total Carbohydrate 9g, Dietary Fiber 2.1g, Total Sugars 4.3g, Protein 2.1g

Raspberry Lemon Muffins

Prep time: 15 min Cooking Time: 15 min serve: 2

Ingredients

½ tablespoon plain yogurt

1 tablespoon coconut oil

½ tablespoon lemon juice

1 egg white

½ teaspoon lemon extract

½ cup flax meal

½ tablespoon honey

¼ teaspoon baking powder

¼ teaspoon salt

1/8 teaspoon grated lemon zest

1 tablespoon frozen raspberries

1 cup water

Instructions

In a large bowl, mix the yogurt, coconut oil, lemon juice, egg white and lemon extract. In a separate bowl, stir together the flax meal, honey, baking powder, salt, and lemon zest. Add the wet ingredients to the dry, and mix until just blended. Gently stir in the frozen raspberries. Spoon batter evenly into the prepared muffin cups.

Pour 1 cup water into the Instant Pot. Place the trivet inside. Place the muffin cups on the rack or pan.

Secure the lid and set the Pressure Release valve to Sealing. Press the Pressure Cook or Manual button and set the cook time to 20 minutes.

When the Instant Pot beeps, allow the pressure to release naturally for 10 minutes, then carefully switch the Pressure Release valve to Venting. When fully released, open the lid. Carefully remove the muffins.

Nutrition Facts

Calories 123, Total Fat 8.5g, Saturated Fat 3g, Cholesterol 0mg , Sodium 158mg, Total Carbohydrate

Blackberry Peach Muffins

Prep time: 15 min Cooking Time: 20 min serve: 2

Ingredients

½ cup coconut flour

1 tablespoon honey

½ teaspoon baking powder

1 pinch salt

1 egg

¼ cup coconut milk

½ tablespoon melted butter

¼ cup blackberries

1/8 cup peeled and diced fresh peaches

¼ teaspoon ground cinnamon

1/8 teaspoon ground nutmeg

1 cup water

Instructions

In a large bowl, stir together the coconut flour, honey, baking powder and salt. In a separate bowl, mix the egg, coconut milk, cinnamon, nutmeg and ½ cup of melted butter until well blended. Pour the wet ingredients into the dry, and mix until just blended. Fold in the blackberries and peaches. Fill muffin cups with batter.

Pour 1 cup water into the Instant Pot. Place the trivet inside. Place the muffin cups on the rack or pan.

Secure the lid and set the Pressure Release valve to Sealing. Press the Pressure Cook or Manual button and set the cook time to 20 minutes.

When the Instant Pot beeps, allow the pressure to release naturally for 10 minutes, then carefully switch the Pressure Release valve to Venting. When fully released, open the lid. Carefully remove the muffins.

Nutrition Facts

Calories 145, Total Fat 7.7g, Saturated Fat 5.4g, Cholesterol 45mg, Sodium 68mg, Total Carbohydrate 16.9g, Dietary Fiber 7g, Total Sugars 5.6g, Protein 3.9g

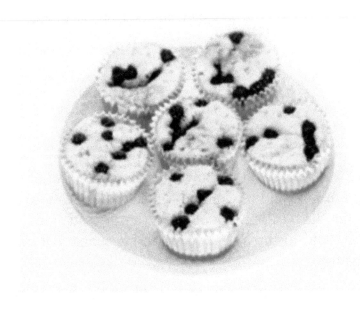

No-bake keto granola bars with peanut butter

No-bake keto granola bars peanut butter, easy healthy granola bars. Creamy peanut butter, flaxseed meal, chia seeds, almonds, coconut and more! 100% Sugar free, gluten free paleo breakfast or snacks.

Prep Time: 10 mins Total Time: 30 mins

Servings: 8 breakfast bars

Ingredients

Wet ingredients

1/2 cup Natural Peanut butter or almond butter if paleo 1/4 cup Coconut oil

2 teaspoons Vanilla extract Dry ingredients

1/3 cup Erythritol - like erythritol

1/2 cup Sliced almonds + extra 1 tablespoon to decorate on top 1/3 cup Flaxseed meal

1 tablespoon Chia seeds 1/3 cup Pumpkin seeds

1/4 cup Unsweetened desiccated Coconut 1/2 teaspoon Cinnamon

Chocolate drizzle

3 tablespoons Sugar-free Chocolate Chips 1 teaspoon Coconut oil

Instructions

Line a loaf pan, size 9 inches x 5 inches, with parchment paper. Set aside.

In a medium mixing bowl or a saucepan, place all the wet ingredients: peanut butter, coconut oil, and vanilla.

Microwave by 30 seconds burst, stir and repeat until the coconut oil is fully melted and combines with the nut butter. It should not take more than 1 minute 30 seconds. Otherwise, melt the ingredients in a saucepan under medium heat, stirring often to prevent the mixture from sticking to the pan.

Stir in the sugar-free crystal sweetener, stir and microwave an extra 30 seconds to incorporate well. Erythritol doesn't dissolve very well but it will give some delicious sweet crunch into your bars or see paleo note.

In a large mixing bowl, add the rest of the dry ingredients: sliced almonds, flaxseed meal, chia seeds, pumpkin seeds, shredded coconut, and cinnamon. Stir to combine.

Pour the nut butter mixture onto the dry ingredients. Stir with a spatula to combine. You want to cover all the dry ingredients with the nut butter mixture.

Transfer the mixture into the prepared loaf pan. Press evenly the mixture with your hand to leave no air. Flatten the surface with a spatula.

Freeze for 20 minutes until the breakfast bars are hard and set. Remove from the freezer, lift the parchment paper to pull out the bar from the loaf pan. Place on a plate. Sprinkle extra sliced almonds on top.

In a small bowl, microwave the sugar-free dark chocolate and coconut oil until fully melted.

Drizzle the melted chocolate on top of the bar, return into the freezer 1-3 minutes until the chocolate is set.

Cut into 8 breakfast bars.

Wrap each bar individually into plastic wrap or bee wax. Store in the fridge up to 8 days.

Nutrition Info

Calories 306 Calories from Fat 253 Fat 28.1g Carbohydrates 9.6g Fiber 6.8g Sugar 1.4g Protein 7.9g Net Carbs 2.8g

Pecan Pie Muffins

Prep time: 15 min Cooking Time: 25 min serve: 2

Ingredients

1 tablespoon honey

1 cup coconut flour

1 tablespoon chopped pecans

1tablespoon butter, softened

1 egg, beaten

1 cup water

Instructions

In a medium bowl, stir together honey, coconut flour and pecans. In a separate bowl beat the butter and egg together until smooth, stir into the dry ingredients until combined. Spoon the batter into the prepared muffin cups.

Pour 1 cup water into the Instant Pot. Place the trivet inside. Place the muffin cups on the rack or pan.

Secure the lid and set the Pressure Release valve to Sealing. Press the Pressure Cook or Manual button and set the cook time to 25 minutes.

When the Instant Pot beeps, allow the pressure to release naturally for 10 minutes, then carefully switch the Pressure Release valve to Venting. When fully released, open the lid. Carefully remove the muffins.

Nutrition Facts

Calories 97, Total Fat 7g, Saturated Fat 2.9g, Cholesterol 49mg, Sodium 44mg, Total Carbohydrate

6.9g, Dietary Fiber 1.6g , Total Sugars 4.8g, Protein 2.3g

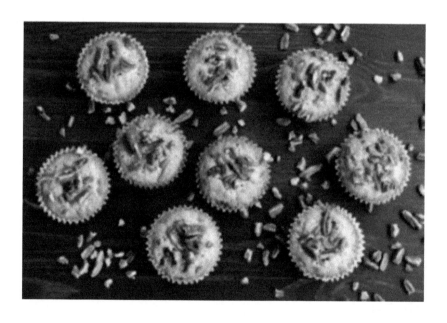

Spinach-Egg Muffins

Prep time: 10 min Cooking Time: 25 min serve: 2

Ingredients

1 cup spinach, chopped

2 eggs

¼ teaspoon salt

¼ teaspoon freshly ground black pepper

¼ teaspoon coconut oil

½ large white onion, chopped

1 cup water

Instructions

In a large bowl, whisk the eggs together and add the salt and pepper. Set aside.

In a pan, heat the coconut oil and sauté the onion until translucent for 3-5 minutes. Remove from the heat. Add the onion and spinach to the eggs and mix well.

Pour 1 cup water into the Instant Pot. Place the trivet inside. Place the muffin cups on the rack or pan.

Secure the lid and set the Pressure Release valve to Sealing. Press the Pressure Cook or Manual button and set the cook time to 20 minutes.

When the Instant Pot beeps, allow the pressure to release naturally for 10 minutes, then carefully switch the Pressure Release valve to Venting. When fully released, open the lid. Carefully remove the muffins.

Nutrition Facts

Calories 125, Total Fat 5.8g, Saturated Fat 2g, Cholesterol 164mg, Sodium 446mg, Total Carbohydrate 8.4g, Dietary Fiber 4.3g , Total Sugars 2.4g, Protein 9.8g

Crispy Tofu

Prep time: 5 min Cooking Time: 15 min serve: 2

Ingredients

1 cup tofu, cut into pieces for your choice

Salt and freshly-cracked black pepper

1 tablespoon butter

½ cup tomato sauce

½ tablespoon lime juice

Chopped fresh cilantro

Instructions

In a medium mixing bowl, whisk together the tomato sauce, lime juice combined. Set aside until ready to use.

Season tofu pieces on all sides with salt and pepper.

Click the ─Sauté‖ setting on theInstant Pot . Add the butter, followed tofu, turning every 45-60 seconds or so, until the tofu is browned on all sides. Transfer tofu to a separate clean plate, and repeat with the remaining tofu, searing until it has browned on all sides. Press ─Cancel‖ to turn off the heat.

Pour in the tomato sauce mixer, and toss briefly to combine with the tofu. Close lid securely and set vent to — Sealing

Cook on high pressure for 2 minutes, followed by a natural release (about 15 minutes).

Sprinkle with chopped fresh cilantro, then serve and enjoy.

Nutrition Facts

Calories 171, Total Fat 11.2g, Saturated Fat 4.8g, Cholesterol 15mg, Sodium 382mg, Total Carbohydrate 6.7g, Dietary Fiber 2.4g , Total Sugars 3.6g, Protein 11.4g

Plum Skillet Cake

Prep time: 15 min Cooking Time: 50 min serve: 2

Ingredients

2½ tablespoon coconut oil

½ cup almond flour

¼ teaspoon salt

¼ teaspoon baking powder

1/8 teaspoon baking soda

2 tablespoon honey

1 large egg

½ cup low-fat buttermilk

2 medium ripe plums, pitted and thinly sliced

2 tablespoons coconut sugar

Instructions

Butter an 8-inch cast iron or oven-proof skillet. Dust with flour, tapping out any excess.

Whisk together almond flour, salt, baking powder, and baking soda in a medium bowl.

Combine coconut oil and honey in a large bowl; beat with an electric mixer on medium speed until pale and fluffy. Beat in egg. Add flour mixture in 3 batches, alternating with buttermilk, beating batter briefly after each addition.

Pour batter into the prepared skillet and smooth the top with an offset spatula. Fan plum slices on top of batter, and sprinkle with remaining coconut sugar.

Pour 1 cup water into the Instant Pot and arrange the handled trivet on the bottom. Place the pan on top of the trivet and cover it with an upside-down plate or another piece of parchment to protect the brownies from condensation.

Secure the lid and move the steam release valve to Sealing. Select Manual/Pressure Cook to cook on high pressure for 45 minutes. When the cooking cycle is complete, let the pressure naturally release for 10 minutes, then move the steam release valve to Venting to release any remaining pressure. When the floating valve drops, remove the lid.

Let cool slightly before serving.

Nutrition Facts

Calories 396, Total Fat 37.3g, Saturated Fat 31.4g, Cholesterol 48mg, Sodium 236mg, Total Carbohydrate 14.4g, Dietary Fiber 0.5g, Total Sugars 13.7g, Protein 2.9g

Yellow Squash Brownies

Prep time: 15 min Cooking Time: 45 min serve: 2

Ingredients

1 tablespoons coconut oil

½ tablespoons honey

½ teaspoon vanilla extract

1 cup coconut flour

½ tablespoon unsweetened cocoa powder

½ teaspoon baking soda

1/8 teaspoon salt

1 cup shredded yellow squash

¼ cup chopped walnuts

Instructions

Grease and flour a 9x13-inch baking pan.

In a large bowl, mix the coconut oil, honey and 2 teaspoons vanilla until well blended. Combine the coconut flour, cocoa, baking soda and salt; stir into the honey mixture. Fold in the yellow squash and walnuts. Spread evenly into the prepared pan.

Pour 1 cup water into the Instant Pot and arrange the handled trivet on the bottom. Place the pan on top of the trivet and cover it with an upside-down plate or another piece of parchment to protect the brownies from condensation.

Secure the lid and move the steam release valve to Sealing. Select Manual/Pressure Cook to cook on high pressure for 45 minutes. When the cooking cycle is complete, let the pressure naturally release for 10 minutes, then move the steam release valve to Venting to release any remaining pressure. When the floating valve drops, remove the lid.

Let cool slightly before serving.

Nutrition Facts

Calories 108, Total Fat 8.7g, Saturated Fat 3.8g, Cholesterol 0mg, Sodium 243mg, Total Carbohydrate

6.3g, Dietary Fiber 2.3g, Total Sugars 3.1g, Protein 2.9g

Apple Pie Quinoa Pudding

Prep time: 5 min Cooking Time: 10 min serve: 2

Ingredients

2 cups quinoa

2 cups apples finely chopped

1 cup soy milk

½ tablespoon cinnamon powder

½ tablespoon Vanilla free

1/8 teaspoon ground cardamom

½ cup golden dates

Instructions

Place all Ingredients in the Instant Pot.

Cook on manual at high pressure for 10 minutes. When time is up, quickly release the pressure.

Serve and enjoy! This is delicious served hot, warm or cold.

Nutrition Facts

Calories 251, Total Fat 2.7g, Saturated Fat 0.3g, Cholesterol 0mg , Sodium 34mg, Total Carbohydrate 50.5g, Dietary Fiber 6.8g, Total Sugars 28.4g, Protein 5.9g

Baked Peaches

Prep time: 10 min Cooking Time: 15 min serve: 2

Ingredients

1/8 cup apricots

1/8 cup dates chopped

1/8 cup walnuts chopped

1 teaspoon nutmeg

1 tablespoon honey

4 small peaches

2 tablespoons coconut oil

1 cup Water

Instructions

In a small bowl, mix apricots, dates, walnuts, nutmeg and honey.

Using a paring knife, remove the peaches cores, leaving the bottom 1/2 inch of the peaches.

Fill apples with filling mixture and top each with a thin slice of butter.

Pour 2/3 cup water in the Instant Pot and arrange the apples in the bottom of the pot. Add any extra butter to the cooking water.

Secure the lid, making sure the vent is closed.

Use the display panel to select the Manual or Pressure Cook function. Use the + /- keys and program the Instant Pot for 3 minutes.

When the time is up, let the pressure naturally release for 5 minutes, quickly releasing the remaining pressure.

Serve warm.

Nutrition Facts

Calories 299, Total Fat 14.9g, Saturated Fat 12.1g, Cholesterol 0mg, Sodium 4mg, Total Carbohydrate

38.3g, Dietary Fiber 5g , Total Sugars 37.8g, Protein 3g

Simple White Cake

Prep time: 10 min Cooking Time: 30 min serve: 2

Ingredients

1 tablespoon coconut sugar

½ tablespoon coconut oil

1 egg

1/8 teaspoon vanilla extract

½ cup coconut flour

½ teaspoon baking powder

1/8 cup coconut milk

Instructions

Grease and flour a 9x9-inch pan or line a muffin pan with paper liners.

In a medium bowl, cream together the coconut sugar and coconut oil. Beat in the egg, one at a time, then stir in the vanilla. Combine coconut flour and baking powder, add to the creamed mixture and mix well. Finally stir in the milk until batter is smooth. Pour or spoon batter into the prepared pan.

Pour 1 cup water into the Instant Pot and arrange the handled trivet on the bottom. Place the pan on top of the trivet and cover it with an upside-down plate or another piece of parchment to protect the brownies from condensation.

Secure the lid and move the steam release valve to Sealing. Select Manual/Pressure Cook to cook on high pressure for 30 minutes. When the cooking cycle is complete, let the pressure naturally release for 10 minutes, then move the steam release valve to Venting to release any remaining pressure. When the floating valve drops, remove the lid.

Let cool slightly before serving

Nutrition Facts

Calories 260, Total Fat 12.2g,Saturated Fat 8.8g, Cholesterol 82mg, Sodium 54mg, Total Carbohydrate 31.1g, Dietary Fiber 12.4g , Total Sugars 0.7g, Protein 7.6g

Brazil nuts Cake

Prep time: 05 min Cooking Time: 40 min serve: 2

Ingredients

1-1/2 tablespoons sugar-free chocolate chips

2 tablespoons butter melted

1 egg

1 cup all-purpose flour

½ tablespoon arrowroot powder

½ teaspoon baking powder

½ teaspoon pumpkin purée organic

¼ cup honey

¼ cup Brazil nuts, chopped

¼ cup coconut cream

½ teaspoon allspice

¼ teaspoon vanilla extract

Instruction

In a large bowl, thoroughly mix all ingredients, until a perfectly even mixture is obtained.

Next, pour 1 cup filtered water into the Instant Pot and insert the trivet.

Transfer the mixture from the bowl into a well-greased, Instant Pot– friendly pan.

Using a sling if desired, place the pan onto the trivet, and cover loosely with aluminium foil. Close the lid, set the pressure release to Sealing, and select Manual/Pressure Cook. Set the Instant Pot to 40 minutes on high pressure, and

Once cooked, let the pressure naturally disperse from the Instant Pot for about 10 minutes, then carefully switch the pressure release to Venting.

Open the Instant Pot and remove the pan. Allow to cool completely before serving. Serve, and enjoy!

Nutrition Facts

Calories 470, Total Fat 10g, Saturated Fat 7.1g, Cholesterol 82mg, Sodium 40mg, Total Carbohydrate

85.5g, Dietary Fiber 2.6g, Total Sugars 36.2g, Protein 10.1g

Oatmeal Raisin Cookies

Prep time: 15 min Cooking Time: 20 min serve: 2

Ingredients

1 tablespoon coconut oil

1 tablespoon honey

1 egg

1/8 teaspoon vanilla extract

1cup coconut flour

1/8 teaspoon baking soda

1/8 teaspoon ground nutmeg

1/8 teaspoon salt

1 cup rolled oats

1 tablespoon raisins

Instructions

In large bowl, cream together coconut oil, honey, until smooth.

Beat in the egg and vanilla until fluffy. Stir together coconut flour, baking soda, nutmeg, and salt. Gradually beat into butter mixture.

Stir in oats and raisins. Drop by teaspoon complete onto ungreased cookie sheets.

1 cup filtered water into the Instant Pot and insert the trivet.

Transfer the mixture from the bowl into a well-greased, Instant Pot– friendly pan.

Using a sling if desired, place the pan onto the trivet, Close the lid, set the pressure release to Sealing, and select Manual/Pressure Cook. Set the Instant Pot to 20 minutes on High pressure, and

Once cooked, let the pressure naturally disperse from the Instant Pot for about 10 minutes, then carefully switch the pressure release to Venting.

Nutrition Facts

Calories 273, Total Fat 8.9g, Saturated Fat 5.5g, Cholesterol 41mg, Sodium 129mg, Total Carbohydrate

40.1g, Dietary Fiber 14.2g , Total Sugars 6g, Protein 8.2g

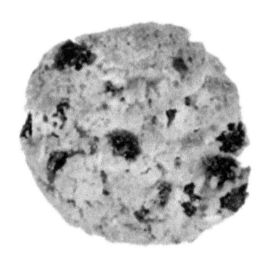

Lightning Source UK Ltd.
Milton Keynes UK
UKHW020755220421
382425UK00006B/74